This Could be The way the Wedding Ended:

A Positive Perspective on Sustaining Partnerships

By

Ronald V. Stanhope

Copyright © by Ronald V Stanhope 2022. All reserved. No part of this book may be reproduce or use in any manner without written permission of the copyright owner except for the use of quotations of the book review.

TABLE OF CONTENS

Introduction

Marriage is not a magical, eternal bond; rather, it is an organic one. Nothing in the statement "till death splits the parties" suggests that a marriage will end. A fact is not the same as an intention. Genesis and the rest of the Bible teach that marriage is what it should be, not that it is an irreversible connection. Sin modifies reality. People don't keep their word. Too many marriages end before they should. A covenant, or agreement between two individuals, is what marriage is: it is a set of explicit or implicit duties that each partner has to the other. Marriage is not an ill-defined, hazy bond. In terms of relationships, people can promise a variety of things to one another, but some necessities must be committed in accordance with God's given morals. These are essentially the man's essential bodily supplies. He is not allowed to physically mistreat his spouse, either by hitting her or by denying her access to necessities like food, clothes, and sex, which allows her to have children for security. She, however, is required to make a sexual allegiance vow to her spouse (monogamy). Additionally, an implied commitment to be together exists. Resigning suggests that the pledges are rejected. In a marriage, two people make these promises to one another with the hope of being together until death separates them. Sometimes a married couple dissolves their union before one of the spouses passes away. Whenever one of the spouses consciously violates one of the fundamental vows, there is a sundering. God provided guidance on the course of therapy. of violators of covenants. The offending lady and her boyfriend faced the death penalty for breaking the wife's fidelity pledge. When a husband violates his commitment to provide physical abuse, whether by or through passive or active means, the outraged woman is liberated from the marriage. A kind of the latter was divorced in a dishonest manner. we discovered that divorce became more of a disciplinary issue in the divine economy. The previous purpose of divorce under the law—namely, to protect women who have been abused—was not really altered by this role enlargement. It adopted a disciplinary role in the prophets. However, the goal of carrying out this disciplinary duty was to bring back lawful marriages.

This book will teach you basic techniques on how to preserve your marriage and triumph over divorce.

Chapter 1
REASONS FOR DIVORCE

On the other hand, some problems that are common among couples heading toward Splitsville include disagreement, adultery, inadequate communication, incompatibility, and a lack of romantic intimacy or sex. Some studies have examined easily quantifiable variables that increase the likelihood of divorce, such as the age at which people marry.

The most significant indicator of whether your marriage will last is how you resolve conflict." Nobody considers nasty arguments, continual strife, and nightly arguments before bed to be signs of a happy marriage.

How long could you endure when the location that should be your haven from the everyday grind and source of calm is really more stressful than your worst day at work? In a happy union, your partner is your closest companion, your storm shelter, and your biggest supporter during difficult times.

Your spouse is just as emotionally harmful in a high-conflict marriage as an awful boss. If therapy or marriage counseling is not used to break this downward cycle, it will continue until divorce is the only option left.

Top 10 Frequent Causes of Divorce.
1. Adultery outside of marriage or having affairs.
Being betrayed by someone who promised to be devoted to you forever is a terrible pill to swallow, and most people don't think it's a crime that can be forgiven. Although adultery doesn't always result in divorce, it certainly ruins your perception of your union.

You have three inquiries when you find out that your husband has been having an extramarital affair:

Will my union endure this betrayal?

Can I ever again trust my partner or spouse?

Will I put forth the effort to improve my marriage, or has my partner's adultery been the final straw?

The answers to these queries will rely on how eager and capable you both are to mend your bond, most likely with a marriage and family therapist's assistance.

In order to save your relationship, you will need to forgive your spouse, and they will need to apologize sincerely and promise to stop cheating going forward. If you've been straying from each other, put more effort into getting back together than assigning blame.

2. A lack of closeness, either physically or emotionally.

Physical and emotional closeness "greases the wheels." of an easy-going partnership. But when they leave, major problems in relationships frequently replace them.

Some of the most serious problems include communication breakdown, anger, resentment, melancholy, loneliness, adultery, and very low self-esteem. If these problems are not addressed, they can cause irreversible harm to a relationship and lead to divorce.

Your sexual life will most likely deteriorate when there is little to no emotional closeness. Your union may turn into a sexless one if you feel emotionally cut off from your partner. attempt to recall the reasons you fell in love with your partner and deliberately attempt to see them through those glasses to rekindle the flame.

Additionally, consider the activities you two used to like doing and schedule time to engage in those activities. Rebuilding emotional connection via time spent doing something you both like might pave the way for physical intimacy.
Intimacy, both physically and emotionally, is like super glue when it comes to securing your marriage and love.

3. Issues in Communication Between Partners.
One of the most important indicators of divorce is a communication breakdown. In contrast to couples that have learned how to politely handle disagreement, poorly communicating couples are unable to work through problems jointly and are more likely to have misunderstandings and upset feelings.
Both verbal and physical communication are essential for practically all aspects of a healthy relationship, including sex, money matters, having children or not, resolving conflicts, and other delicate subjects that unhappy couples feel are too risky to discuss. Lack of communication destroys closeness, love, and respect in a relationship by converting problem-solving sessions into yelling battles. You must be willing and able to discuss what's wrong or not working in order to come up with a solution as a team in order to get through the inevitable difficult periods.

Dr. Edward Dreyfus, a clinical psychologist and life coach, states that effective communication involves both strong receptive (hearing) and transmission (articulation) abilities. Without both, the dialogue will be challenging at best.

4. Abuse by Parents or Partners: Known as Domestic Violence.

Domestic violence encompasses any act of real or threatened a buse, including physical, psychological, sexual, emotional, and fi nancial abuse.. In a relationship like this, one person acquires or keeps control over their relationship via a history of violent conduct.

This abuse may be committed against one spouse only, or it may also affect one or more of the married children.

5. Differing morals or values.

There have been actual conflicts over disparities in race, religion, country, and culture, as well as persecution due to these distinctions combined with gender, sexual orientation, and even political affiliation.

Divorce is likely to result from a marriage between two people who have different morals and/or beliefs and who are unable or unwilling to see things from their spouse's perspective.

He thinks life begins at conception, whereas she supports a woman's freedom of choice; his closest buddy identifies as homosexual, while his wife is homophobic; they fell in love

Despite their differences in religion, they are still in love, but now that they have kids, those differences are destroying them. Red indicators indicating your principles and underlying beliefs are too dissimilar for a successful partnership are often ignored or rationalized when you're in love, but when the rose-colored glasses fall off, those disparities make it difficult or impossible to maintain a happy marriage.

6. Alcoholism: Drug, Alcohol, Gambling, Sexual Addiction. Addiction comes in a wide range of forms and intensities, and many successful professionals—including politicians, executives, physicians, attorneys, portfolio managers, actors, and athletes—have been able to effectively conceal their addiction while rising to the top.

Their partners can be obligingly ignorant, prepared to turn a blind eye in exchange for lifestyle or financial advantages, or are duped into thinking it's insane to worry about their spouse's addiction. The moment of truth is always devastating, regardless of how it arrives.

The capacity and readiness of the addict to accept responsibility for their addiction, their sincere desire to seek treatment, and their commitment to recovery for the rest of their lives will all play a role in whether or not the marriage can last.

7. The lack of romantic love or intimacy.

With how hectic and demanding our lives can be, this one is all too typical. It becomes even more prevalent when you include having to drive the kids to before- and after-school practices for sports like hockey, baseball, ballet, symphony, theater, and chorus.

Too many times, partners put everything else before their relationships, so when one of them declares, "I want a divorce," the other is caught off guard. Unlike what many people think, passionate love is Not self-sustaining: Love withers away like a plant without water or sunlight if you don't set aside time for intimacy and enjoyment as a partnership, not simply as a family.

Establish a weekly dating night that is set in stone. For instance, get up or go to bed earlier and take advantage of the extra time for regular emotional and physical connection, such as hugging or having sex. Before it's too late, think back to the activities you enjoyed doing while you were courting, and get back to those!

8. One spouse is not contributing enough to the marriage.
We've all been in partnerships where one partner works full-time and handles all domestic tasks, food shopping, cooking, and childrearing.

The partner whose job never ends when they come home might gradually build up a strong animosity between one another, and the marriage may end in divorce if the issue is not resolved.

Make a list of everything that has to get done to maintain the household's smooth operation when you sit down. Next, assign a name to each task, making sure to distribute the work fairly. Remember to put your kids' names on chores they can assist with or handle as they become older, such as cleaning the carpets, mowing the grass, washing the dishes, and setting the table.

"Not carrying your weight" also applies to intimacy and romance; if one person is the sole one setting up date nights, planning romantic gestures, or starting sex, it will also negatively impact the marriage.

9. Debt and Money Issues.

 For the past few years, many couples have struggled financially. Divorce may result from a couple's inability to communicate well enough to address their financial issues in a cool, collected manner. Financial arguments can turn bitter and spiteful.

Financial difficulties in a marriage can take many forms, beyond simply being deeply in debt and/or unable to pay for essentials. Couples who have fundamentally different perspectives on money and debt—regardless of how much or little they really own—may find their marriage disintegrating.

If your primary concern is money, you might choose to see a specialist in financial divorce matters. They might suggest the most cost-effective methods for dividing up property, paying taxes, and helping concerns.

10. Incompatibility or lack of shared interests between partners.

It's true that opposites do attract, but commonalities are the glue. If you and your spouse don't have common interests, you'll either find yourself spending less and less time together as you follow your passions and hobbies or you'll give them up in favor of your partner's interests.

These two tactics will erode your relationship and cause you to become resentful. You will probably need to attend marriage therapy and be prepared to make concessions if you want to stay together.

For instance, if he likes bowling and she enjoys dancing, he may go bowling with his friends on Thursdays while she goes out dancing with her pals. After that, they could decide on a "Friday date night" activity that they both enjoy.

That pertains to everything in your joint life, from taking care of the house to deciding which extracurricular activities their kids will participate in. Divorce may result from your incompatibility if you are unable to come to a mutually agreeable settlement.

Chapter 2
EVEN GOOD PEOPLE CAN MAKE BAD PARTNERS

One of the most significant choices you will make in life is whether or not to get married. It necessitates a significant commitment made for the appropriate reasons by the right two individuals.

I'm assuming that if you're reading this, you want to spend the rest of your life—not just a few days or months—with a wonderful guy or woman.

Of course, flings and casual partnerships are perfectly acceptable. However, if you're hoping for anything more committed, like a marriage or a move-in, you should be on the lookout for warning indications that she won't make a good wife.

In the early stages of a relationship, it is easy to be taken by surprise. The majority of individuals admit to witnessing their relationship through rose-colored glasses and come to regret their choice after a few years.

Jokes about how a man changes after he gets married or how a woman changes after she gets married are utterly ridiculous.

People do change, but they don't really shift into someone else. To help you save time and money, it is therefore essential to recognize the warning indications of a lousy spouse early on in the relationship.

It's acceptable if you and your spouse have different views on money, but having completely different financial beliefs strains your relationship. Different financial beliefs can lead to everyday struggles because there are countless financial decisions made in daily life.

While it's common (and even beneficial) for couples to have some intense Well-worded conversations on finances are indicative of a good partnership; once again, effective communication is essential. "Couples should talk about the importance of money in their life, its significance, and the symbols it represents. When it comes to their weekly spending habits, couples nearly never agree and may argue or get into "fair fights" over them. Financial arguments don't have to break you up as long as you're making an effort to communicate and find a middle ground.

Say. The justifications and justifications don't stack up. You could have come upon enigmatic bar tabs, secret bank accounts, or questionable emails. Alternatively, perhaps every day seems like a confusing maze where you can't seem to find a way out. A trail of ambiguity emerges. They either gaslight you or divert your attention when you try to get clarification, or maybe face a potential indiscretion, and then they react by remaining silent and refusing to address your worries.

"Successful weddings are characterized by a solid partnership built on authentic and reliable interaction.

Eight red flags of an unsatisfactory spouse.

1. Issues with commitment.

Getting married is a lifetime commitment.

You make a commitment to your spouse to be there for them through good times and bad. It's quite significant. ·

Consider the commitment level of your potential bride before deciding to commit.

Does your spouse work at many jobs intermittently? Is her best friend always switching every few weeks or months?

It is a definite thing. indication that your significant other is not eager to commit to a long-term relationship.

While there's nothing wrong with being in that phase of life when you're experimenting to find who you are, it's not the stage you want your future spouse to be in when you tie the wedding. It was shown that commitment accounts for 85% of divorces, with arguments coming in second (61%).

When someone can't even plan what they're going to do the following week, how can you plan a life with them?

2. He/she forces you to transform.

How frequently does your prospective partner make you feel self-conscious?

If you find yourself sidestepping this inquiry or using flimsy justifications, do let us know that your partner isn't the right person for you. Your spouse should love you for who you are, after all.

Yes, you want your spouse to eat well and take care of herself, so she can politely urge you to work out or have a salad when she sees you scarping down junk food.

But if all they want to do is try to alter your personality or looks, it's a clue that you two aren't going to be happy together.

And after a few years of marriage, when everything would be really chaotic and convoluted, one or both of you would understand this.

3. An egocentric spouse.

This holds true for relationships in general as well as marriage.

Any kind of Both parties must be willing to compromise and show thoughtfulness in order to maintain a long-term engagement.

Even if you may be a wonderful partner who indulges all of his whims and desires, does your partner reciprocate?

Does your partner have self-interest as their first concern?

If so, there will be severe marital conflict.

Recognize that, upon marriage, you become equal partners and, without further ado, you must look out for one another. Nothing will drive you two apart more quickly than resentment if you don't have the same level of reciprocity.

Even on first dates, it's usually simple to see whether someone is only interested in themselves.

When you witness something like that again, you should make a phone call. It gives up.

4. indulges in excessive partying.

A person who enjoys parties should not be judged negatively, however, some people are extreme party animals.

The majority of ladies who enjoy partying go out three days a week, drink, and have a good time, but they are aware that their social calendar may alter after they get married.

Unfortunately, some women fail to recognize that they aren't prepared for the transition in time.

Thus, before saying "I do," you might want to give it some serious thought if you are the type of person who prefers calm beverages, enjoys long walks and a beautiful setting for dates, and is always juggling clubs.

The majority of males desire to spend a respectable sum of routine spend time with their wives. Yes, you and she are free to go out and have fun with your own groups of friends on occasion.

However, it indicates that she isn't ready to be in anyone's life if she would rather spend time with you than dance the night away with strangers.

It's totally okay if she still likes going to parties like a college student, but you don't want to be that husband who has to convince his wife to remain at home so you can spend some time together.

5. Serious Trust Concerns.

There's no getting around it: trust is one of the most crucial components of a long-lasting, wholesome relationship.

When there is a lack of trust between you, the whole relationship would like you're treading carefully.

When she is your girlfriend, she doesn't trust you. Does she ask how you and your friends are doing, and does she call you out on lying to her?

That won't alter after you are married, though.

Even if you've been the most devoted and faithful person on the earth, a ring on her finger won't make her trust you.

When you haven't even established fundamentals like trust, you can't possibly go down the aisle!

6. Attempts to disconnect you.

Has your partner advised you to avoid specific people?

It can be someone you've known for 20 years as your best friend or your neighbor. Your relatives could even be involved. A spouse acts in a like way when he or she typically anticipates that you would give them your entire life and neglect all other relationships. It's one of the most obvious—and unavoidable—bad marital indicators.

Although your marriage should be one of the most significant partnerships in your life, this does not imply that you should sever all links with others. False!

It won't be your partner who asks you to cut ties with these individuals. Rather, they will gently separate you from your loved ones by playing tricks on you and sowing little doubt-seeds.

 requesting that you "prove" your love for him/her by picking them over them.

Alternatively, they could come up with plans to "permit" or keep you apart from your loved ones. once every several months or years for you to meet them. under their direction, naturally.

You've been duped if you find yourself unable to socialize with anyone and are unable to identify why.

7. causes you to feel self-conscious.

Because they are human, your spouse will err and say hurtful things when they are upset.

Nevertheless, they are ultimately meant to be your largest ally and most reliable source of assistance.

They ought to care for you, encourage you, and foster your growth by giving you a sense of worth and affection.

They ought to support you, particularly at times when it seems like everything is against you.

If your prospective spouse consistently exhibits You're self-conscious, and such remarks are telltale indications of a toxic marriage.

Why would you want the person closest to you to constantly make you feel bad? The world is already pretty dreadful, after all.

Thus, you may wish to take action if you have seen terrible spouse indications in your existing relationship.

8. Doesn't give each other enough time.

One of the most important components of a good relationship is spending quality time with one's partner. It is not a good indicator and the relationship is likely to become one-sided if your partner is not considerate of the time they spend with you, or worse, avoids you.

Your respective worldviews and ideals diverge. It can be worldly interests. opinions, faith, or anything else. One indication that your spouse is not a good fit for you may be if your hobbies do not coincide or if they do not take the initiative to do so.

Chapter 3
WHAT IS IMPORTANT AND WHAT ISN'T

Which ethnicity do you belong to? French, Indonesian, Korean, Papua New Guinean, Nicaraguan?

Which color are you—brown, black, white, or yellow?

Are you tall or short, physically fit or not?

Are you wearing rags or a suit and tie?

It doesn't really matter if you're a president, corporate tycoon, cabinet minister, or regular person.

No, it doesn't matter (on the values scale). It either doesn't matter at all or matters very little for any of them.

The heart is what counts most of all.

How large it is, how flexible it is, and if it's only physical or whether it's more than that;

Whether it is able to connect with the mind or has mastered the ability to soar to the farthest reaches of the planet.

Material goods: Many wise people have stated, and I wholeheartedly agree, that the majority of the stress in our everyday lives is from our material belongings. It gets much worse with modern technology (and the need to keep up with it). Your phone cracked, your car's radiator failed, you can't install USB drivers, or your pricey massage chair requires service. You don't even know it when your possessions start to rule your everyday existence. You would be so much more content and liberated if you didn't have to worry about constantly buying, maintaining, and getting rid of stuff. While I'm not promoting extreme austerity, my point is that Windows 98 is still functional.

Ego:

You are the main cause of stress in your life.

The depressive state brought on by failing to pass the exam, the fixation with (financially) outdoing friends, neighbors, and class mates, and the obsessional urge to prove oneself right (and oth ers wrong), the arguments over the wrong shade of blue paint on the wall, and the rage over a friend losing your favorite book are all examples of this. It's also acceptable to travel by bus or taxi, not own that fancy car, even if you don't have a phone (or have a bad network provider, like mine, MTNL). This freedom from material possessions makes you feel like a free bird without any heavy baggage. It's not society or the other person you are at odds with in these instances; it's you. Do these petty ego battles really matter in the long run? Are these ego battles, which leave you or the other person feeling horrible, improving your life? Isn't it better for everyone if you start placing less value on yourself? Even though it can be difficult, try living a day when you don't care about yourself. Your life will be a lot more fulfilling because you'll be able to put your ego aside and concentrate on the things that truly count in life.

Experiences:

 Living a life full of new experiences is one of the greatest things about being alive. Experiences revitalize, educate, and thrill you. In contrast to tangible belongings, the Photographs, tales, and recollections of these moments won't fade and don't need to be maintained. Have you ever considered taking a global travel tour? Do it if not! The budget is not a limitation. Take a language course. Take a bungee leap. Take a rideshare. Launch a brand-new charitable venture. Taste some novel, unusual foods. You may immerse yourself in literally millions of various kinds of experiences, the majority of which don't need a large financial investment. Typically, your ego keeps you from experiencing new things and, as a result, keeps you from growing as a person and experiencing life to the fullest. This happens under the false pretext that you are preoccupied with the routine of everyday life. These encounters are most beneficial since they allow you to interact with several fascinating individuals, some of whom may possibly wind up being longtime companions and friends. Developing and preserving connections with your parents, friends, siblings, spouses, kids, and even neighbors is one of life's most fulfilling experiences. To be happy and maintain their sanity, humans require other humans. A recluse can quickly go insane. Unfortunately, though, sometimes our ego causes us to be hasty in these interactions and we wind up doing harm to others. Understanding that the ties you have with other people are far more essential than yourself is crucial since even ignoring them might result in loneliness or broken relationships (this insight is for your own benefit and contentment, given your reliance on others. Attempt living by yourself!). Joy and happiness only seem true when shared with others, don't they? Is it possible to be content by yourself? Not at all! So set aside your ego and work to make your connections stronger. Make sure you have someone to tell about your experiences from your vacation to the Caribbean when you get back (and no, I don't mean your Facebook buddies)

Chapter 4
DECEPTION AND SEX

Living as though falsehoods were the truth, a marriage or a relationship with a loved one, but once the truth is embraced, the effects of living lies start to heal.

Nothing compares to having a companion with whom you completely trust and have complete faith. You are aware that they are sincere, devoted, and loyal, and that they will always support you. You share everything, both the wonderful and unpleasant things that happen in between your everyday lives together. You converse about everything. A relationship where you conceal information from your spouse or even tell what you would consider to be "little white lies" is the reverse of this kind of trusting connection. I refer to them as falsehoods, or more accurately, as deadly tiny white lies. Nothing can sabotage your relationship more quickly than lying and secrecy. Any kind of deception kills confidence.

Fear is the main source of these small white lies. You lie to your spouse or withhold information out of fear that they may become irate if you explain everything. You rationalize this by claiming that you are defending both your relationship and your spouse. This has the potential to turn into a self-destructive habit or even an addicting game. The excitement of surprising your significant other with something, or the joy of acting illegally while fooling yourself that you're not damaging anything. Little lies are the beginning of this kind of conduct, but even they may damage your relationship when (not if, when) sabotage your relationship more quickly than lying and secrecy. Lying in a way that gets exposed. Like with any form of deceit, you eventually find yourself in a situation where you have to lie repeatedly to cover up your prior lies until you are in a very difficult situation. Then, what do you do?

People's misconceptions about sex in marriage are one of its worst enemies. They still suffer from inhibition and have the incorrect mindset, yet they want and crave more sex.

1. Dirty and terrible is sex.

Though well-intentioned Christians say this to shield us from the sin and suffering of premarital sex, our relationship suffers when we carry that mentality into our marriages.

In actuality, God created sex, and sex is excellent. Sex is a lovely, pure, and God-honoring act of love within a married relationship.

God loves marital sex so much that He wrote a whole book on it in the Bible. God gave married couples the gift of sex, saying, "Eat, friends, and drink; drink your fill of love" Some teach that having sex is terrible and disgusting, whereas popular culture claims that having sex is only physical. We would like to think that obtaining physical fulfillment may be achieved without causing emotional or spiritual harm.

In actuality, sex is a private conversation that unites two individuals. During intercourse, chemicals like oxytocin are produced in the brain to strengthen the emotional relationship between the partners. Our friendship gets stronger the more we work together. However, it gets more difficult to build that connection with the next person the more individuals we do it with. God created sex for marriage for this reason. We unite on a physical, emotional, and spiritual level during sexual activity.

2. What happens next when two people fall in love?

If intimacy unites us, isn't that what happens when two individuals fall in love?

The fact is that having sex outside of God's plan is lustful, not loving. Seeking what's best for the other person is a selfless act of love. Lust is the self-centered pursuit of what will satisfy me right now.

God intended for marriage to be a beautiful display of love via sex. Having sex before being married, even for a few weeks or days, is the desire and deception of The one we love and we are harmed by God's creation.

Sex is really lovely, and the best kind of sex can only be had according to the manufacturer's instructions. Almighty.

See for yourself how wonderful and significant sex is by reading the Song of Songs!

3. I'm not getting my gratification.

The Truth: Delaying sex until after marriage will increase your enjoyment significantly!

Everything that God made, including sex, is excellent.

You can't escape sex. However, everything that is utilized improperly turns into abuse, and abuse is never attractive. You may have pleasure with your spouse in your married bed without having to share it with anybody else if you save sex for marriage. Marital sex is incredibly lovely, thrilling, and enjoyable.

Aside from union, "Let the marital bed become clean, and let marriage be regarded in esteem among all, for God will judge the sexually unlawful and illicit," is a is a statement that still feels good in the here and now.

5. Sex desire is destroyed by religiosity. It's not sinful or bad, your spouse. Engage your partner in meaningful and personal conversations to elevate your sexual life to a thrilling new level.

Chapter 5
MARRIAGE: WAYS TO AVOID DIVORCEMENT

Divorce is unavoidable in certain cases. The divorce card is the last one you should play, though, if you're still in love and in a committed partnership. Without a doubt, saving a marriage is a superior play, especially if you know how to accomplish it.

If you and your spouse don't intentionally make adjustments to improve the situation, things can quickly spiral out of control once they start to go south.

1. Put Your Relationship First.

It is not unusual for people to begin to believe that the grass is greener on the other side when things are difficult. Even the notion that you could be happier outside of your marriage might seriously strain your relationship—even if you never say what's on your mind.

It might be more difficult to dedicate yourself to your partner when you dwell on what your life would be like if you weren't married. It may also deplete your motivation to work on strengthening your union.

Make up your mind in advance that divorce is not an option in order to minimize the risk to your partnership. By making the commitment, you'll be able to stop worrying about what life could be like after marriage and instead concentrate on strengthening your relationship.

2. Pardon Immediately

Resentment from one partner is a common reason why marriages fail. Studies have indicated that harboring disdain for your spouse nearly invariably lingers and, if left unresolved, can result in divorce.

Forgiveness is among the most crucial and the hardest things for couples to accomplish, when couples forgive each other, they can move forward because forgiveness is a window that allows To look earlier in desire to remain mired within side the painful times that when befell them."

As soon as you can, try to forgive your lover. Recall that self-forgiveness is an equally valuable gift. Keeping a grudge requires mental and emotional room, and it usually has a negative effect on your stress levels and general well-being.

3. Have the Will to Say Sorry.

Ask for your partner's forgiveness and provide a heartfelt apology if you have offended them. Pay attention to what they say and make an effort to comprehend, what is upsetting them. Inform them that you plan to work on doing things in a different way going forward.

4. Show your partner respect and honor.

Individuals will always change with time. Any connection must be able to comprehend, value, and adjust to such changes. To remind yourself of the amazing person you married, start by compiling a list of all the nice things about your spouse. You can recollect your initial feelings for them by doing this activity. Expressing your gratitude for your partner's peculiarities and oddities can also be beneficial.

Tell your partner how much you appreciate all they do every day by giving them praise or saying "thank you."

These little words are equivalent to bank deposits. It is not advisable for you to leave your marriage without never having placed a deposit. Therefore, make sure that everything you do respects your spouse for who they are.

5. Keep In Touch Frequently.

With the prevalence of Smartphone's, Netflix, and remote work, it's simple to become sidetracked in this day and age. You may discover that you frequently go days without speaking with your partner in person."Couples who communicate often are able to express their emotions and let go of past hurts. Grudges frequently start when one person believes their other diminishes their feelings and does not listen to them.

6. Discuss Your Expectations for Money.
Money disputes are a common source of stress in relationships.7. Different financial expectations are frequently brought to a relationship by couples. It may be challenging for each spouse to view the financial status from the other's point of view.
deciding on how your finances are managed is a vital part of a happy marriage. Decide on a spending plan, a debt management strategy, and a way to live within your means. Making the distinction between necessities and wants is also crucial. Although both are acceptable, couples may run into issues if they attempt to satisfy every need without taking their budget into account.
Budget flexibly so that you may cover presents, entertainment, getaways, and other things that can improve your marriage.

7. Allow each other some room.
Determining the ideal amount of time to spend together is one of the most difficult things to balance in a marriage. While too

little might be perceived as inattentive, too much can be oppressive.

When your spouse requires time alone or a night out To make sure they can obtain that time, volunteer to watch the kids or run errands with pals. However, you should also schedule time for your relationship. If you can't find someone to watch the kids or you have limited funds, organize a fun and affordable date night at home.

The important thing is that you both intentionally try to spend time together and give each other room to have separate lives.

8. Put wellness first.

It's simple to get into an excessively casual habit, particularly after a long relationship. Thinking back to your initial dating experiences might help you revive the romance: getting ready for a date night by getting a manicure at home, having a new haircut and shaving, or dressing up for pleasure.

There are several methods to feel energizing and appealing. Maintaining your physical health improves your mood and self-esteem.

Whether you're preparing healthy meals together, trying out a new fitness class, or training for a 5K, it may also serve as a chance to spend quality time with your significant other.

9. Enjoy Date Evenings.

Courting your spouse is another strategy to keep the spark alive in a marriage.10 Schedule a date night once a week, even if it's only to grab ice cream or try a new dish.

Spending quality time together is crucial. "Spending quality time together as a pair involves going out and sharing, which helps to fight monotony, enables individuals to enjoy themselves more as a pair and get to know each other better.

If cost is an issue, think about exchanging babysitting duties with another couple that wants to go on a date night.

Alternatively, you might just stroll the infant around the mall or go to the neighborhood park.

Maintain your dating routine by engaging in the same activities. Thoughtful, little acts may make a pair feel like newlyweds.

Consider making their favorite food at the grocery store, placing small love notes where they will find them, or making them coffee in the morning.

10. Avoid Trying to Manage Your Spouse.

Both spouses respect one another and don't push for their personal interests in a happy marriage. This may signify various things to different couples, however, the following fundamental ideas should be kept in mind:

Avoid attempting to supervise or manage one another.

Allow your companion to be themselves without restriction.

When making important decisions, learn to work together (such as spending money and parenting children)

Give your spouse permission to come and depart without requesting it from you.

There is a hazard that controlling companions will become emotional abusers. They may exhibit indicators of financial abuse, which often results in divorce.

11. Seek Assistance.

If your marriage is still not working out or you think a divorce is coming soon, think about getting counseling or couples therapy.

 This can be a beneficial approach to solving issues you may be having and acquiring new abilities that will make your marriage stronger

Seeing a psychologist can assist them in developing new goals as a married couple, improving their relationship, and efficiently resolving issues.

12. Shut up and pay attention.

We had been given one mouth and ears for a reason. In certain situations, talking too much might be likened to throwing gasoline on a fire. When the cause of combustion is eliminated, the flame will go out, allowing you both to gather your thoughts and reconsider your strategy to solve the difficulties at hand.

Fearful or furious spouses will often take out their frustrations on their partner and make sure they have their way. At times, though, their only want is to vent, and that will alleviate their discomfort. Allowing your partner to speak things out while you stay quiet and pay attention is one method to resolve conflicts. The secret, of course, is to keep your eyes open.

Being silent and attentive is one thing, but tuning someone out while they are sharing their deepest thoughts is quite another. When you don't put in enough effort, trying to do the right thing might turn into doing the wrong thing at that point.

13. Order your priorities anew.

Your marriage must be your first focus if you want to keep it together when it's in danger. This entails giving it precedence over your kids, your work, or anything else that demands your attention.

It's not meant to suggest that you should ignore everything else as doing so would only lead to marital dissatisfaction; instead, prioritize your relationship above all else in your life.

Rather than spending a Saturday night out with the girls, grabbing drinks with the men to watch another game, shopping, escaping for the day to run errands, or engaging in any other leisure activity, resolve to dedicate time to your marriage.

You don't have to go crazy, but you should make sure your partner understands that they are once again the center of your attention.

Another advantage of doing this when you have children is that those acts also relieve their tension and provide them with a clear sign that their parents love one another.

14. Give up being so rude.

You are aware of the subject at hand. While each one of the tiny exchanges that make up a marriage won't end it, when combined, they can cause a great deal of animosity.

Making insensitive remarks about someone else's appearance or demeanor, failing to remember to buy the right groceries, shoving the kids away from your partner when you know you should be involved in whatever is happening, purposefully not answering your phone, critiquing their cooking, using excessive sarcasm, making inappropriate jokes or joking, calling your spouse fat, and so on and on and on it goes.

This is sometimes caused by cruel or self-centered behavior rather than the kind of unconditional love that is the foundation of happy relationships.

It's inevitable that you may receive some criticism, but learn to take it personally and only respond appropriately when it's appropriate. Play the MIA card only when absolutely necessary. Be in contact early and often.

Don't vent your frustrations on the one person who should be your greatest ally when you're having a rough day. Instead, tell them what's upsetting you or that you're in a funk. Ask for assistance. Additionally, you must also take a step forward while the other shoe is on it. Provide at least as much as you take.

15. Take care of your addictions.

Too many people use drink and drugs to dull the hurt of a failing relationship. If you must immerse yourself in your sadness, do it sparingly.

Even the strongest marriage can be swiftly undermined if one partner has an extremely severe addiction that they are unable to control. If you find yourself in that situation, consider if you want to continue dancing with those demons or return to the original reason you were drawn to your partner.

Remember that in many states, addictions to drugs or alcohol may be used against you if they play a role in your final divorce. They might be quite influential on matters pertaining to child visitation, alimony, and asset partition. Should your dependency be excessive enough, you can most effective be capable of see youngsters beneathneath supervision, or possibly now no longer at all. Your marriage might be destroyed by other harmful habits as well. Addictions to porn or shopping can sometimes cause serious problems in a marriage. Seek treatment if you have an addictive personality before it ruins your marriage and your life as a whole.

Conclusion
THE PROCESS OF REACHING TOMORROW

Everyone wants to love and be loved, no matter where they live. For the majority of our lives, we hunt for the ideal mate. They become one in marriage when you believe you've discovered the one and are prepared to spend eternity together. However, some unions end in divorce because of the two parties' failure. Divorce rates have been rising in today's culture throughout time. The church is becoming less dogmatic, marriage is viewed as temporary, and there is no reason why divorce rules force couples to remain together. The resolution Whether or not both parties should divorce depends on their respective expectations and worldviews. The real secret to a happy marriage is foundation and dedication. When there is violence, contempt, infidelity, and a breakdown in communication, a marriage is not committed. Without the power of mutual commitment, relationships cannot advance. Love cannot exist when there is disrespect. It is simple for spouses to be open, secure, and connected to one another when there is respect. Infidelity and abuse undermine respect in a partnership and lead to its dissolution. Nobody should continue to be physically or emotionally mistreated and cheated on in a relationship. If someone feels compelled to lie, they are clearly unhappy in the partnership. When one partner is away looking for attention from others, the marriage cannot progress. Love is the foundation of marriage, and love has no bounds. Never mistake faithfulness and cruelty for love. Remember that love is never going to harm you, even if you feel that you are in love. A lack of loyalty is a lack of respect. Marriage shouldn't be seen as a passing phase because it lasts forever. A small disagreement here and there can always be resolved. There's a distinction between disagreement and never-ending combat. Never accept less and never believe that being abused or cheated on in a marriage is acceptable. Once an abuser, constantly an abuser, and as soon as a cheater, constantly a cheater.